MW01141618

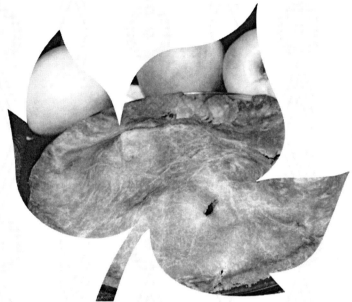

ILHENAYLH
"feast"

YVONNE WYSS

amy,

Enjoy in good Health

Yvonne

Copyright © 2014 by Yvonne Wyss
First Edition – June 2014

ISBN
978-1-4602-3975-9 (Hardcover)
978-1-4602-3976-6 (Paperback)
978-1-4602-3977-3 (eBook)

All rights reserved.

No part of this publication may be reproduced in any form, or by any means, electronic or mechanical, including photocopying, recording, or any information browsing, storage, or retrieval system, without permission in writing from the publisher.

Author Photo by Glenda Monsen.

Produced by:

FriesenPress
Suite 300 – 852 Fort Street
Victoria, BC, Canada V8W 1H8

www.friesenpress.com

Distributed to the trade by The Ingram Book Company

TABLE OF CONTENTS

Dedication iii

Origins v

How It All Began . . .
The Journey to Traditional Living vii

Measures xi

Gluten-Free Flours xii

    Almond xii

    Coconut xii

    Corn xii

    Fava Bean, Other Beans xiii

    Quinoa xiii

    Rice xiii

    Sorghum xiv

    Tapioca xiv

    Teff xiv

Thickeners, Binders, Substitutions, and Other Additions xvi

    Guar Gum xvi

    Buttermilk xvii

    Gluten xvii

    Coconut Oil xvii

    Olive Oil xviii

    Walnut Oil xviii

    Vinegar xix

    Sugars xix

    Spices xx

Gluten-Free Flour Blends xxi

Gluten-Free Signature Blend xxi

Kloshe Sapolill House Blend xxii

Historical Points of Interest xxiii

Deer Roast with Mock Mashed Potatoes 3

Bison Tourtière 5

Bison Shepherd's Pie 8

Bonnie's Chicken and Turkey Strips and Wings 10

Salmon Cakes 12

Barbecued Salmon 14

Fish and Chips 16

Broth 18

Bison Soup 20

Chicken Soup 22

Pizza 24

Wild Rice Stuffing 27

Fried Wild Rice 29

Mac 'n' Cheese 32

Bannock 34

Flaky Buttermilk Biscuits 36

Hamburger and Hotdog Buns 38

Tortillas 40

Historical Points of Interest 41

Pancakes 45

Strawberry Sauce 47

Squamish Bars 49

Coffee Cake 52

Cinnamon Buns 55

Banana Bread 59

Fresh Fruit Pie 61

Pie Crust 63

Regular Homemade Pie Crust 65

Almond Coconut Tart 67

Carrot Cake with Cream Cheese Icing 69

All-Occasion Cake 71

Coconut Power Bars 74

Herbal Teas 79
    Chamomile 79
    Dandelion 79
    Elderflower 80
    Fennel 80
    Labrador 80
    Lavender Flower 80
    Lemon Balm 80
    Nettle 80
    Peppermint 81
    Raspberry Leaf 81
    Rose Hip 81
    Rosemary 81
    Thyme 81

Bibliography 83
    Used for research on oils and fats. 83

This book is designed to provide helpful information on gluten-free foods, recipes, and cooking. It is not meant to be used, nor should it be used, to diagnose or treat any medical condition. For diagnosis or treatment of any medical problem, consult your own physician. The publisher and author are not responsible for any specific health or allergy needs that may require medical supervision, and are not liable for any damages or negative consequences resulting from any treatment, action, application, or preparation to any person reading or following the information in this book. References are provided for informational purposes only and do not constitute endorsement of any websites or other sources. Readers should be aware that the websites listed in this book may change.

Education is the key in the world of gluten free! Read your labels and understand what you are buying. Fewer ingredients are always the best option. The less processing, the better. If you are not sure what an ingredient is, then research until you gain a better understanding of it. And keep in mind that natural does not always equal good for you!

DEDICATION

This book is dedicated to those special people who have journeyed with me throughout my life, shaping my passion for food, cooking, and gluten-free healthy living.

My Partner Ken Drury — You have inspired me to stretch my horizons on food and have renewed my outlook on how we fuel and look after the machines we call our bodies. Thank you for eating all my burnt offerings and appreciating and trying everything with enthusiasm and kindness. You are my hero.

My children Tasha, Nicklaus, Brandon, and Tyler, and my stepson Riel — You have been long on tolerance and huge on appetite, putting up with and supporting my many trials and errors in creating these recipes. Thank you all for your honest opinions about what is good and what sucks!

My mother — I remember being a little girl and asking you to teach me to bake pies like Granny. I harassed you until you taught me how to make pastry dough. You were stunned—though you couldn't bake a pie to save your life, you could explain the process perfectly! Thank you for being an amazing teacher.

My father — When I was a child, you were the chief cook in our family. Using your expertise as a meatcutter, you taught me how to clean and can fish, and showed me how to preserve vegetables and fruit. You brought your Swiss influence and your passion for hunting and fishing to my life, as well as an appreciation of our country and its wildlife. My own love of the outdoors reflects your bright influence, and with gratitude, I raise my hands to you now. Thank you for instilling me with such wonderful teachings.

My granny – My earliest memories are of you taking your pies to sell at the Mosquito Creek Marina. What a very industrious woman you always were, finding ways to feed your large family of nine children. You cooked, cleaned, and worked hard. I know what that is like. I am driven that way too. You could say that it is in my blood. Thank you for setting such a fine example.

My other mother Nancy – You have helped me refine my cooking and baking skills, and I love sharing recipes with you. Thank you for teaching me to appreciate all cultures and their food.

My uncle Maurice – You shared with me how and why the concept of ilhenaylh is important to our people, and your teachings are invaluable. Huychewx! Miigwetch! Thank you!

ORIGINS

Health and wellness include the physical, mental, spiritual, emotional cultural, environmental, social, and economic well-being of you, your family, your community, your nation . . . and all your relations!

—Elder's wisdom, *Berry Cakes*

Ilhenaylh (ill-hen-ail) means "feast" in the Squamish language. As an Aboriginal Woman a descendant of the Squamish and Sto:lo First Nations people of British Columbia on the West Coast of Canada, I have found the concept behind this age-old tradition to have tremendous influence on the way I view and prepare food.

My people, the Squamish, have always made sure to cook extra food for guests. We never want to be short of food for our family and friends, because they have been generous to give of their time to be with us. This custom goes back to a time when people would travel great distances by canoe or on foot to attend ceremonial gatherings or celebrations. Food would always be ready for them to take back on their journey home. Generosity and hospitality continue to be among the greatest values held by the Squamish people.

The Squamish believe it is important to prepare oneself in a good way when planning to invite people to share a meal and their time. Being in a positive frame of mind is essential when preparing and cooking food, because, in turn, the food is infused with all these prayers and heartfelt thoughts. This acts as a blessing for guests. At the same token, negative or bad feelings can go into the food as well and make guests sick physically or spiritually.

Aboriginal philosophy teaches that health equals not only freedom from disease, but also a robust body, mind, and spirit. Thus, through experience and the teachings of their elders, succeeding Native generations have learned to select foods in proper amounts to supply the body with the required nutrients. Food is not only a source of energy and vitality, but also medicine.

Historically speaking, plant and animal life were considered sacred by the Squamish and therefore never to be wasted or taken unnecessarily. There was a strongly held belief that the Creator provided food for everyone, so each person had a duty to share his or her food with others. This relationship was often expressed through legends and daily customs. Thus, this cookbook contains teachings and anecdotes pertaining to the legends and daily food customs cultivated over a period of two hundred years by Squamish First Nations people. These can be viewed as snippets of indigenous wisdom geared toward offering cultural perspective and encouraging overall balance in lifestyle and health.

By highlighting dietary changes that have arisen from the consumption of traditional to more modern foods, this book seeks ways to blend both categories through gluten-free cooking, something that is especially close to my heart.

How It All Began . . .
The Journey to Traditional Living

I write this book with the hope of leaving an impression on people why it is important to change how we look at food. Gluten free living is not about cutting things out – it is about changing the way you eat and look at food. This book is written from my world view as an Aboriginal Woman living in Canada and all the experiences it includes. I live Within the Lower Mainland of British Columbia lies the Traditional territory of Skwxwu7mesh Uxumixw (Squamish Nation). I would like to share some of my culture through the medium of food.

Throughout the book there are teaching sections which will offer you options for living healthier, balanced way of life. My perspective is from a cultural and spiritual view, so I view food as medicine as much as I do nutrition. I am mindful when I am preparing food as we contribute energy for us all is connected in the circle of life.

Some time ago, I ended up in Abbotsford Regional Hospital in British Columbia suffering from kidney failure, myocarditis, pneumonia, and pleurisy. For a two and a half month stay, I was at what I jokingly referred to as "the - spa, – where the "food is lousy but the service is awesome." I went to work as soon as I was healthy enough. Through this journey with my health led to my losing over sixty pounds. this due to makingthe dietary changes I made in the food I eat.

As soon as I was healthy enough, I returned to work. This was the first job I had held in over twelve years. It was with Fisheries and Oceans Canada, which was an amazing experience. I had been a stay-at-home mom with my four children, and I moved my family to Ladner, British Columbia. Now, I am a firm believer that life puts one exactly where one needs to be exactly when one needs to be there. This happens so that one can learn an important lesson or meet someone who is meant to play an important role in one's life for a pivotal period of time.

This is why I needed to be in Ladner. So I made the transition. Though the change was somewhat lonely for me, for most of my kids it was fine. They adjusted and managed despite some minor issues. My youngest son, however, had the most difficult time. I discovered his ADHD and just how severe it was. He was to struggle with this and lose an entire year of schooling because of it. Eventually, my son's condition forced my family back to Abbotsford. Regardless, what I learned from this experience was that we could move to a different city and be okay. We survived.

Moving back to Abbotsford was the right thing to do at this time. I ended up finding employment with Corrections Canada, where I would work in the federal prison system with aboriginal offenders. I had finally found something I had a knack for and really enjoyed doing. Despite there being many broken people in the system, I liked working with these guys. This was also where I met the man I am with now. He has a story of his own. Health complications had left him with cancer and allergies that made him change the way he looked at food as well. In fact, he suffered from such severe food allergies that he could not eat most food, the way he had most of his life.

Ken and I would soon spend a lot of time eating together. We'd have lunch at work and often also have meals after work, and we talked a lot about food. I joke that I have never met a man who eats as much as this one! Ken is always eating; he always has a bag of vegetables or fresh fruit. These are the foods that constitute most of our regular diet. People think that it is hard to live the way we do—but it isn't at all. It's not rocket science. It's not unusual or odd. All it takes is a little planning, and it's actually pretty easy once you get the hang of it. Thanks to the changes we made in the way we eat, we are healthier and happier. I lost weight just by eating differently and with no exercise involved. And what's more, I felt better by putting a different kind of fuel into my body.

Ken's lifestyle and choices inspired me to write this book. He opened my eyes to how beneficial gluten-free living could be. I learned to eat the way he does, and I changed my own perspective on food and how to look after myself in a healthier way. Along this journey, we both learned and taught each other a few things. Since childhood, I had always loved spending time in the kitchen—my favourite room in the house—and preparing food. But for a long time, I had lost my inspiration. Ken brought the sunshine back into my life and made me want to cook and bake again. When I look back, it's funny to think that I had forgotten how much I enjoyed cooking.

To this day, our conversations revolve around meals, sustainable living, and how to feed communities and our children. We talk about food as medicine, and as a way of life. Although he underestimates his own accomplishments, Ken is also a terrific cook in his own right. He just lets me cook for him to make me feel better. I suspect he likes to be pampered and fed.

After two years of effort and experimentation, we have figured out how to cook for and feed our family according to tradition. And now, we want to share this way of life with others. We hunt, we utilize and balance what is available to us, and, by planning ahead and bringing what we need, we improvise when we are in a place where there is not a gluten-free store or restaurant available. Packing food to go is essential to us. I encourage the kids to eat before we leave and always pack snacks to travel with. I know how hungry everyone is all the time. It is never an option to be without food!

When my youngest son was diagnosed with ADHD, to the best of my ability, I changed his diet to being almost exclusively gluten free and with almost no processed sugar. He has very few behavioural problems now and his ADHD is manageable. There are, of course, other things that we help him work on as well, but adjusting his food intake was a big factor in turning things around for him. Now he plays hockey and lacrosse and is a healthy little boy who is doing very well! All our kids are benefiting from eating healthier, gluten-free foods. Children are more than capable of making choices about food and educating themselves once they understand how food works and the effects it can have. They are amazing at retaining information when they are engaged in the process.

The path to gluten-free living is different and requires learning a new way of embracing food, but it doesn't necessarily have to be hard. It seems that as awareness of the effects of gluten has increased in recent years, more and more people are taking a closer look at just how gluten might be affecting their lives and the lives of their loved ones. During my own journey, as I educated myself on gluten, I discovered that this protein derived from wheat and related grains can be found in many food products, and sometimes even in those one would never expect to find it in. Many people's bodies cannot adequately process this protein, which explains why it leads to a variety of digestive and other health-related problems, some of which can be severe.

Through experience, I have realized that there is a notable distinction between the separate categories of people who cannot handle gluten. There are people with celiac disease, for example, in which the lining of the intestine becomes damaged due to exposure to gluten, and then there are those with gluten intolerance. Allergies and intolerance are different. I am intolerant, whereas my partner and his son are allergic. What does this mean? It means that they will have allergic reactions, while I will experience discomfort. Either way, by eliminating gluten from our diets as much as possible, we avoid adverse health effects and enjoy better quality of life.

I wrote this book in the hope of helping others achieve the same. Gluten-free living is not about cutting things out; it is about changing the way one eats and looks at food. Please note that because this book has been influenced by experiences that are specific to those within my home, the recipes within are somewhat limited toward what has been successful for my family. But adjustments can be made to suit your preferences and those of your household accordingly.

I hope you enjoy this book, and that it assists you in making healthier choices. May the lives of you and your family parallel the positive experiences of mine.

Miigwetch! Thank you!
Yvonne

MEASURES

lb = pound
kg = kilogram
Q = quart
L = litre
C = cup
oz = ounce
T = tablespoon
t = teaspoon
g = gram

Adjustments for Recipes in Other Provinces

Please note that the liquid measures and cooking temperatures listed for my recipes are based on my location in British Columbia. It is important to remember that if you live in another province, you must make the appropriate adjustments to achieve the best results. As a veteran cook and baker, I can tell you that this is necessary because altitude and air pressure affect recipes. For example, if you are located in Manitoba, you will need to add almost an additional three-fourths to a full cup of water to your pancake batter in order to get the same consistency. Allow for more baking time as well for cakes and other similar items, and make sure to do your toothpick tests prior to removing your baked goods from the oven so that they are properly cooked through.

Gluten-Free Flours

Almond

Almond meal is a very expensive but great option for baking. It adds wonderful flavour and texture. I use this extensively in crumbles, bars, squares, tarts, and crusts for pies.

Coconut

Coconut flour is used for baking and has a terrific smell, but it is very spongy and requires a lot of liquid to work with. It is not well suited for binding, though it has a great flavour and is good in small amounts for blending. Though it is not my preference to use coconut flour in my baking, I do use other forms of coconut, such as oil, nectar, and sugar. These are all wonderful products that are low in glycemic value and high in fibre, nutrients, and other vitamins. I do, however, purchase a terrific coconut bread made with only coconut flour, coconut, salt, and water that is absolutely amazing and the only bread used in my home!

Corn

This is not the best alternative in my home because of its generally high level of processing and additives. I might use corn chips, for example, but not cornstarch. So I use tapioca instead, as it is less likely to cause allergic reactions in my family members. I have used corn flour, but only in limited quantities.

GMO is a term tossed around today and not necessarily defined. This abbreviation stands for "genetically modified organism." The majority of corn today is genetically modified unless otherwise specified as being organic, and the latter is not always readily available. Corn is a crop that is used in everything from fuel to medication. A source of controversy, it is nevertheless cheap to produce, is versatile, and is thus heavily funded by the government and supported by big companies. Through my research, I have found that corn is not as gluten free or as safe for those with gluten intolerance as we are led to believe, either. One has to be careful in seeking out information about what is safe to use.

FAVA BEAN, OTHER BEANS

Bean flours are widely used in gluten-free cooking. They are good sources of protein, even in small amounts, as well as stable additions to blends. Some have an aftertaste. Many commercial blends of flours have some type of bean flour in their blends. They are reasonably priced and readily available, but may not be the best option for people with gas and intestinal issues.

QUINOA

This is a complete protein. It has an even flavour that is slightly nutty. In small quantities in a blend, it provides stability and protein needed for nutrition. It's great for breads and biscuits. Small amounts are good for using in bars and squares. I use quinoa in the following forms: flakes, seeds, and flour. I use it as a complete protein for cooking and baking, adding it to puddings, stir-fry dishes, and flours. This ancient grain is an all-around source of nutrition that gets a lot of regular use in my home.

RICE

Wild rice, sweet rice, brown rice—there are many. Be mindful of your choices, though, as some have flavours that you may not want in your baking. For example, wild rice is strong and dark in flavour and colour, and is great for gravies and soups.

Sorghum

Also known as *Sorghum bicolor*, this is a species of grass. It is grown mainly in Africa, Central America, and South Asia. Cultivated for its grain, which is widely used in poor and rural villages, it is a major world crop that is also utilized for making "syrup," molasses, and alcoholic beverages. Sorghum is considered one of the five most important food crops in the world. I use it in flour form in high quantities in my own flour blends.

Tapioca

This is used as a starch. In the starch form, it adds no flavour for use in cooking gravies, bars, squares—just about everything. I use it as a staple in all my cooking. As a granulated crystal, it is perfect for making fruit jams, pies, and compotes. Tapioca thickens, but does not affect colour or clarity in fruit, nor does it add any flavour.

Teff

This is one of the smallest ancient grains. From a grass family similar to sorghum, teff grows on long stems also referred to as lovegrass. It is native to northeast Africa and southwestern Arabia, and has long been widely used in Ethiopia. The seeds are so tiny that they are easily lost, and the word "teff" itself means "lost" in the Amharic language.

Teff flour is a dark, heavy flour I mix in small quantities into my flour blends. It adds a high fibre content. In addition, this small grain gives the body three main types of energy: fast release, slow release, and endurance. Its nutritional value is phenomenal. It aids in muscle building and tissue repair, and provides calcium, magnesium, and vital minerals and vitamins for growth.

Teaching

In my personal journey and experimentations, I have found that the best way to be confident with gluten-free flours is to take a recipe you are really familiar with and adjust it with a gluten-free substitute until you are happy with the results. By using your own recipe you can make adjustments until it works to your liking. It is like chemistry—try and try again until you succeed!

I spent two and a half years creating a flour blend that has the closest consistency to the gluten alternative and is perfect for all-purpose substitution in all recipes. This blend also has a neutral taste that does not overpower cakes, shortbread cookies, or any other delicate desserts. It rises well in yeast breads and in regular baking. It is also a terrific alternative to thickeners for making gravy and sauces. The Kloshe Sapolill flour blend I use throughout is thus well researched and tested.

THICKENERS, BINDERS, SUBSTITUTIONS, AND OTHER ADDITIONS

GUAR GUM

A type of polysaccharide, guar gum is the ground endosperm of guar beans. It allows binding, is a powerful thickening agent, and has almost eight times the elasticity of cornstarch. The only downside I see for this product is that it falls under the classification of a bean. So if you have difficulties with bean-based items, you might want to stick with xanthan gum.

Xanthan Gum

This gum is a polysaccharide, a carbohydrate secreted by the bacterium *Xanthomonas campestris*. It was discovered by Allene Rosalind Jeanes and her research team at the United States Department of Agriculture in the 1950s, and has been widely used since the 1960s in the food industry as a food-thickening agent. Check ingredient lists on products at the grocery store just for fun and see if you can find it!

A Note on Gums: I sometimes combine guar gum and xanthan gum. When used together, their elasticity and binding potency create a result that is the closest to gluten but without its potential negative effects. Though each can be used on its own, combined they create a more stable product that is better for baking and consistency. In this case I use equal parts xanthan and guar gums.

If you have four cups total of gluten-free flours, then add one teaspoon of either combined gums or just the one you prefer for every cup of flour. But keep in mind that some recipes ask for less of the gums. This is why I tend to add gums later when I am baking and to blend my flours without the gums, as I am never sure of what gum levels are required for a specific recipe. Pizza utilizes a higher gum content due to the need for dough elasticity, for example. Conversely, biscuits need less gum to bind them and keep them fluffy and airy. Bars and squares need little or no gum at all to make them crumbly and melty. So choose and apply your gum combination when you bake rather than putting it into your blend first.

BUTTERMILK

To make my version of buttermilk, add one teaspoon of lemon juice to one cup of soy, coconut, or almond milk and let stand for a couple of minutes. Traditional buttermilk is a soured milk culture, and lemon juice creates the chemical reaction needed for this. I use alternatives to cow's milk due to the lactose issues in my home. My kids don't notice a difference in any dishes I prepare with this buttermilk recipe, so I think it is quite comparable to traditional buttermilk.

GLUTEN

This is a composite protein that for some people does not break down in the body and that subsequently causes problems in those with gluten intolerance. Because it is not properly processed, gluten builds up in the body and causes things like "leaky gut." It is a binding agent that provides the lovely, fluffy stickiness found in regular flour and flour-based foods. All but one recipe in this book completely exclude gluten.

COCONUT OIL

A personal favourite in my home, this versatile oil contains lauric acid (a saturated fat found in breast milk) and has many health benefits, such as lowering HDL cholesterol in the blood, making it a good option for diabetics. It can restore normal thyroid function, which is important for overall body function. And it helps fight off viral and bacterial infections, and fungal infections, including those caused by candida. By adding this wonder oil to your normal diet, you can significantly boost your immune system.

OLIVE OIL

Many properties in olive oil are believed to promote good health. Oleocanthal, a phytonutrient, is said to mimic ibuprofen and assist in reducing inflammation. Squalene, which aids in biosynthesis, and lignans, a class of antioxidants, are other positive attributes of olive oil. It is low in saturated fat, high in antioxidants, and contains carotenoids, which are good for protecting against UV rays. I use extra virgin cold pressed, the oil that is extracted during the first pressing and is of the highest and purest quality.

WALNUT OIL

Though it is starting to become more popular, this oil is expensive and hard to obtain. I found it first in a natural food store and then of all places at Liquidation World. I use it sparingly and usually only for salads and wild rice pastas once they are at the serving stage. This oil is tasty and offers excellent nutritional value. A real treat!

Earth Balance Butter, Earth Balance Shortening

Both of these products are excellent. I use only the sticks, and not the spread, though this brand makes a coconut spread that is wonderful and amazing! I like to use the shortening sticks for pastries and bannock—it's great for baking. The butter sticks work just as well. You don't need a lot, and these products are good especially if you have family members with vegan preferences, or reactions to other fats and trouble with dairy.

Dough Improver

Here is a simple recipe for a stabilizing gluten-free baking agent:

    2 C (500 ml) granulated soy lecithin or rice lecithin
    1 T ascorbic acid
    1 T ground ginger

Grind the soy or rice lecithin in a food processor or blender until a powdery consistency is achieved. The texture of lecithin is sticky and dry; it feels tacky to the touch. Mix in the ginger and ascorbic acid and store in a dry container. It will keep for months. I use it regularly to stabilize my baking. One to one and a half teaspoons are usually required per recipe.

VINEGAR

It is amazing how many different uses this acid has. It is utilized for preserving and creating everything from sauces to salsa. Vinegar is a no-go in my home because it facilitates yeast growth, so I had to find an alternative: lime juice or lemon juice.

SUGARS

There are so many varieties of sugars. They come in both natural and processed forms, and these can create interesting challenges for diabetics and allergy-sufferers alike. There are up to thirty-seven varieties of sugar produced in the world today across seven different countries. Each has a different glycemic value.

Cane sugar is sucrose extracted from sugarcane and makes up 70 percent of the world's sugar. Brazil is the largest producer of sugarcane in the world. The remaining mass-scale sugar production comes from beet sugar, which is also used for commercial purposes. Coconut sugar and natural fruit sugars like date sugar are other options, as are honey and maple syrup, which are used in many recipes in this book.

Honey is another popularly used sweetener. Its production begins when honeybees collect nectar from plants in the region they live and regurgitate it onto cells in their honeycomb. As these bees add a special enzyme during the regurgitation process, the nectar ripens, its water content evaporates, and honey is formed. It is generally a good option for adults. In fact, honey can boost the immune system. When used in moderation, it can help fight off colds and the flu. Quite literally, an ounce of prevention!

While very tasty, cane sugar can create ulcers and sores for some people, and honey should not be fed to infants, as it can be toxic to their intestinal tracts. So be sure to do your research when deciding what types of sweeteners to use when baking and cooking. All sugars have specific glycemic values, which affects how they are digested and how the body creates insulin, especially in the case of diabetics. For example, processed cane sugar has a glycemic value between eighty and one hundred. Honey has a glycemic value of thirty-one to seventy-eight, depending upon the variety. Coconut sugar has a glycemic value of thirty.

There are many different sugars on the market. However, these types of sugars are the most widely used today and are contained in most products we are familiar with and use in our daily lives. A general rule of thumb with sugars—as with most foods—is, the less processing, the better. Unprocessed sugar is actually more delicious; it has better flavour and offers a healthier alternative for those with a sweet tooth.

SPICES

Herbamare is a spice mixture by Alfred Vogel, a renowned Swiss naturopath. Made with sea salt, celery, leeks, cress, onions, chives, parsley, lovage, garlic, marjoram, rosemary, thyme, and kelp, and free of MSG, gluten, lactose, milk protein, additives, and preservatives, it is an excellent natural product that can be picked up at local grocery stores. This spice mix can be used with most savoury dishes. I use it in many of my recipes. I cook for my elderly parents a lot, and this suits them fine. It is often the only spice I can get my father, who has dementia, to eat.

Vanilla Bean, Extract and Powder: The extract comes in many formats such as pure extract, organic which does not use sugar but uses alcohol and imitation which has additives. The bean can be used and scrapedto etake the vanilla out and then the outer hull can be put in anything you cook to extract the most use of your vanila bean flavour. The powder form of Vanilla bean is the most versatile. This forms is dried and ground vanilla bean and can be added to ll recipes. It is the only version we purchase now and I use it in teas, shakes, baking and all cooking that requires vanilla. Dollar for dollar it is the best use of Vanilla.

Gluten-Free Flour Blends

I have created two gluten-free flour blends that are "all purpose" flours. These blends are versatile and work for all recipes in the book, including those with and without yeast.

Gluten-Free Signature Blend

4 C tapioca flour
3 C potato starch
3 C sorghum flour
2 C quinoa flour
2 C sweet rice flour
1 cup teff flour

Blend and store mixture in a large Tupperware container. Use as needed.

These items can be purchased at local grocery stores such as the Mega Bulk Barn in Abbotsford, Roots in Maple Ridge, and Natural Foods in Mission. The Bulk Barn in Manitoba was a great source for purchasing while my family and I travelled this past summer. Some of the flour ingredients can be found in limited quantities and varieties at Superstore, Save-On-Foods, and IGA. Yields 15 cups.

KLOSHE SAPOLILL HOUSE BLEND

(Chinook trade language for "good flour")

    40% sorghum flour
    35% tapioca starch
    15% quinoa flour
    10% teff flour

Mix all ingredients together and put in a container for storage in the fridge or freezer. It is a good idea to prepare small batches, as gluten-free flours tend to have shorter shelf lives than regular all-purpose flours. Yields vary.

Teaching

Choosing gluten-free flours is about striking a balance. It isn't so much a necessity. Don't get too caught up in the different types of flours—there are so many gluten-free alternatives. What's most important is to pay attention to the ratio for blending and to create blends that appeal to the tastes and needs of you and your family. Blending flours is necessary, as most gluten-free flours have qualities that are not suitable for exclusive use due to their nature. There can be digestion and other related issues. Spend some time researching the flour prior to adding it to the recipes found here. There is a world of information within reach, and personal research is always best to determine individual needs. Trial and error is often still the best way to go. People with sensitivities figure this out only through blending, finding what works, and eliminating whatever doesn't. I am listing only what works in my home; you need to learn what works in yours. Good luck on finding your perfect blend!

Historical Points of Interest

Chief August Jack was well known in the late 1930s as a storyteller and was recorded by Major J. S. Matthews, a city archivist of Vancouver. The following is an excerpt about early Squamish life:

"Whiteman's food change everything," said August Khatsahlano in a conversation while we sat at lunch in a downtown restaurant. "Indians had plenty of food long ago, but I could not do without tea and sugar now. These days Indians who do not want tea and sugar know nothing about it. Lots meat, bear, deer, beaver, cut up meat in strips and dry—no part wasted, not even guts—fill him up with something good, make sausage, just like Whiteman's. Only head wasted; throw head away. Then salmon—plenty salmon. Sturgeon, flounder, trout, lots all sorts fish; come sun-dried; lots crab and clam on beach.

"But Whiteman's food change everything. Everywhere Whiteman goes he change food. China, other places, he always change food where he goes.

"I was born Snauq, the old Indian village under the Burrard Bridge. When I little boy I listen to old people talk. Old people say Indians' first Whitemans near Squamish. When they first see ship they think it an island with three dead trees, might be schooner, might be sloop; two mast and bowsprit, sails tied up. Indian Braves in about twenty canoes come down Squamish River, go see. Get nearer, canoes come down Squamish River, go see. Get nearer, see men on island; men have black clothes with high hat coming to point at top. Think most likely black uniform and great coat turned up collar like priest cowl.

"Whitemans give Indians ship's biscuits; Indian not know what biscuit for. Before Whiteman come Indian have little balls, not very big, roll them along ground, shoot them with bow and arrow for practice, teach young Indian so as not to miss deer. Just the same you use clay pigeon. Indian not know ship's biscuits good to eat, so roll them along ground like little practice balls, shoot at them, break them up."

SAVOURY

DEER ROAST WITH MOCK MASHED POTATOES

Deer Roast:

4 cloves crushed garlic

4 lb deer roast

2 t Herbamare seasoning (or your choice of seasoning)

¼ C fat

olive oil

pepper to taste

salt to taste

Mock Mashed Potatoes:

1 head cauliflower

1 C ricotta cheese

salt to taste

pinch of nutmeg

Boil the cauliflower until it is soft in a large dutch oven pot. Once cooked until completely soft, drain in a colander and return to dutch oven to mash it. Add the ricotta cheese, salt, and nutmeg. Mix until everything is well blended. Use a stick blender if you want to further cream the cauliflower. This dish is low in fat and a nice meal replacement for potatoes.

Turn oven to 350 degrees. Put the deer roast in a roasting pan. I use a clay roasting pan, as this keeps the meat tender and retains heat for roasting. Put the crushed garlic, a bit of olive oil, and salt and pepper to taste on the deer roast. You can also add turmeric, rosemary, and sage. Roast for about three hours. This will cook a 4-pound roast.

Serve with my mock mashed potatoes or with regular potatoes mashed with soy milk, butter, nutmeg, and salt. You can soak your potatoes for 20 minutes in a saltwater brine prior to boiling them to remove some of the starch and reduce the carbohydrate content as well. Make sure you rinse the potatoes and replace the water with clean water prior to boiling. I add a pinch of salt when I replace the water prior to boiling. I do this with my fries. It makes them a lower-calorie potato option.

Preparation time: 25 minutes
Cooking time: 3.5 hours
Serving: 8 servings
Calories per serving: 344

Bison Tourtière

Crust:

Use Pie Crust recipe

Filling:

1 lb ground bison
1 clove crushed garlic
1 t olive oil
1 small-sized onion, finely chopped
1 C peas and carrots
1 t savoury
¼ t ground cloves
¼ C tapioca starch
¼ C water

Preheat oven to 350 degrees.

Fry the onion and garlic in the olive oil. Add the ground bison and cook until browned. Add the spices, cloves, tapioca starch, water, and peas and carrots.

Roll out the pie crust and put it in a pie plate. Fill the pie crust with the cooked meat mixture and put the top crust over it. When I roll out pastry I put the ball of dough between two pieces of parchment paper in order to keep it from sticking to the counter and to make it easier to transfer the pastry to the pie plate. Once it is roled out take the top parchment paper off and place this side down into the pie plate and remove the second piece of parchment paper as you settle the pastry into the pie plate.

Place the pie plate in the oven and bake for 30 minutes, until the top crust has cooked.

Serve with broth as gravy and side vegetables or wild rice.

Double this recipe, as it is a popular and yummy dish and goes fast!

Preparation time: 35 minutes
Cooking time: 20 minutes for meat filling
Baking time: 30 to 45 minutes
Yield: One 9-inch pie
Serving size: 1 piece of a 9 inch pie
Calories per serving: 357

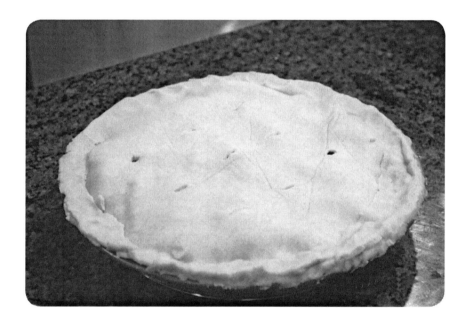

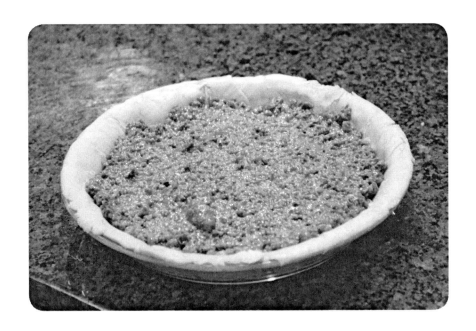

Story Time

Ken once told me a story about how his mom used to make tourtière and how much he missed this traditional dish. I had also grown up with it being served at Christmas. So I went to work coming up with a gluten-free version. Trying my hand at modifying my regular pie crust, I was able to adjust my old recipe to create a flexible and flaky gluten-free option. The next step was to use meat we could eat. For years, I had made tourtière with pork, so for a change, I used ground bison and added the spices and ingredients I had used with pork. I also found I needed to use gravy instead of fat because pork has a lot of fat in it and bison is very lean. This was a great compromise. I now make enough gravy to pour over the tourtière once it is baked. This is a regular meal in our home nowadays.

Bison Shepherd's Pie

Filling:

2 C bison broth (see recipe under Broths)
2 T tapioca starch
1 lb ground bison
1 clove crushed garlic
1 t olive oil
1 medium-sized onion, finely chopped
½ t Herbamare
1 C peas and carrots
pepper to taste - a pinch
salt to taste – a pinch

Topping:

1 head cauliflower
½ C ricotta cheese
½ t salt

Preheat oven to 350 degrees.

Sauté the onion, garlic, olive oil, Herbamare, salt, pepper, and bison together. Add the peas and carrots, tapioca, and broth. Heat until the tapioca is not cloudy and has thickened the broth.

Steam the head of cauliflower until it is soft. Mash it completely and remove all liquid by draining it thoroughly. Add the ricotta cheese and salt. Blend well. Use the same process as the Deer roast and mashed potatoes for cooking and mashing the cauliflower.

Put the meat mixture into a casserole dish. I like to use my stoneware casserole dish. The dimensions are approximately 8" x 4" x 4". Cover the meat mixture with the cauliflower topping.

Put the casserole dish in the oven and bake for 25 minutes. Then turn up the heat to 500 degrees and broil for another 5 minutes, until the cauliflower topping has browned slightly. You can add soy cheese on top if you want a slight variation of this dish.

Preparation time: 25 minutes
Cooking time: 20 minute for cauliflower, shepards pie 30 minutes
Baking time: 30 minutes
Yield: 8 x 4 x 4 dish
Serving size: 1.5 cup serving for 6 servings
Calories per serving: 156

BONNIE'S CHICKEN AND TURKEY STRIPS AND WINGS

2 kg chicken wings
2 kg boneless, skinless chicken thighs
2 C Kloshe Sapolill house blend
1 large boneless, skinless turkey thigh
2 t MSG-free Hy's Seasoning Salt
a dash pepper

Note: I separate the turkey and the chicken onto different baking sheets because of allergy issues in my home. So with that in mind, I also coat the turkey first and the chicken second in the Kloshe Sapolill. If you are really fussy, you can make separate batches of flour mix, but I don't.

Note: if you do not need as much meat adjust the amount of meat you use and make your flour batch ahead and divide before using it to coat your meat.

Preheat oven to 375 degrees. Line two baking sheets with parchment paper. Put the wings on one of the baking sheets and sprinkle them with Himalayan sea salt and pepper. Put them in the oven immediately, before you start the strips. They take longer to cook, about 45 minutes.

Cut the chicken and turkey into about ½-inch strips. Mix together the Hy's Seasoning Salt and the Kloshe Sapolill in a large ziplock bag or a container with a lid that seals so you can shake the strips to coat them thoroughly. Take a handful of strips at a time and completely coat them in the flour and seasoning salt mix. Shake off the excess flour carefully and place the strips on the other parchment-lined baking sheet. Put the strips into the oven.

About 10 minutes into baking, I flip the strips over and brown them on the other side. I use thighs, as they already have some fat in them and the meat is juicier than breast meat. If you use a drier cut of meat, remember to use some kind of fat, and either spray or drop it onto the strips. This will add additional flavour and tenderness. I like to use coconut oil because it has so many health benefits (please refer to the section titled "Thickeners, Binders, Substitutions, and Other Additions").

Fully cooked, the strips should be browned lightly on both sides and not overdone, as this will dry them out. You want them to be juicy and chewy. These are very yummy—in my home, we eat them a couple of times a week, hot or cold! They also travel very well as to-go snacks. I pack them for road trips and whenever my kids go to play sports.

If I may say so myself, these are better than the commercially fried varieties, because mine are healthy *and* tasty!

Preparation time: 15 minutes
Baking time: 45 minutes for the wings
20 minutes for the strips
Yield: 4.5 kg meat or aproximately 9 lbs
Serving size: ¾ lb meat or .75kg per person or 10 servings
Calories per serving: 662

SALMON CAKES

2 T olive oil
2 cans salmon with bones and juice, crushed completely
2 T tapioca starch
1 T fresh or freeze-dried cilantro, finely chopped
1 T fresh or freeze-dried dill
1 egg white
½ C cooked quinoa
½ red or white onion, finely chopped
½ t turmeric
pepper to taste
salt to taste

Note: Used fresh, canned, or smoked, salmon was a very important food among First Nations peoples, especially the Squamish and Sto:lo— my people.

Mix all ingredients together and press into cakes. Add olive oil to a frying pan or a flat griddle and cook until the cakes are golden brown on each side.

It takes about half an hour from start to finish to make these easy, gluten-free, protein-packed salmon cakes. Salmon, of course, is high in omega-3 fatty acids and protein, and the quinoa adds another complete protein—I like to mix red, black, and white quinoa together for texture and taste. Turmeric is a great spice that is high in antifungal properties.

Very nutritional and tasty, this is a great meal when you are in a hurry and need to feed the family fast.

Preparation time: 30 minutes
Cooking time: 10 minutes
Yield: 8 cakes
Serving size: 4 oz with 2 cakes per serving
Calories per serving: 226

Barbecued Salmon

cedar plank(s)
1 filleted side of salmon per plank (approximately 4 lbs)

Note: Salmon grilled on a cedar plank is a common method for preparing this fish. It is also a Squamish tradition.

Place the salmon on the cedar plank(s). Grill the salmon until the white fat of the fish appears evenly over the surface of the fillet. This takes approximately 20 to 25 minutes, depending on the size of the fillet. A 4-pound fillet will take this amount of time. The key is to watch the salmon to ensure it has an even distribution of white. Leaving it to grill for any longer will dry out the salmon. In fact, it is better if the fillet is only partially white at its thickest point.

Cedar planks should be free of any chemical treatments or coatings. They are soaked in water for several hours prior to grilling to prevent burning. Submerging the planks in a baking pan of water works well. They must be weighted down to ensure they soak completely. Salmon fillets should be prepared so that they fit on the planks of cedar. Whole fillets can be placed on longer planks, while shorter ones can be used for salmon steaks. The salmon should be as fresh as possible. Wild salmon has the most flavour, but farm-raised salmon is also acceptable, and less expensive.

Preparation time: 10 minutes
Cooking time: 20 to 25 minutes
Yield: 4 – 1lb servings
Serving size: 1lb
Calories per serving: 85

Story Time

Squamish people also used the "ironwood" bush to cook salmon over an open fire. *Holodiscus discolor*, commonly known as ocean spray, creambush, or ironwood, is a shrub of western North America and is common in the Pacific Northwest, where it is found in both openings and the forest understory at low to moderate elevations.

When my dad came to Canada in the 1960s and met my mom, he was working for Canada Packers as a meatcutter and my mom was working at the fish canneries near Terminal Avenue in Vancouver. My father loved the Native way of life and learned as many of the teachings as he could from my grandfather Lorne Whitton Nahanee and my grandmother Eva Mae Nahanee (Caufield). My grandfather used to get my dad to drive him to Squamish to harvest the ironwood for sticks to cook salmon on. My dad learned what trees to look for, and how to choose the straightest ones, clean them, and prepare them to cook fish on. My dad used to cook salmon this way in a 150-foot open pit for the Salmon Queen Festival in Steveston, British Columbia. He used mostly alder wood to cook with and would get the fires hot with a good base of coals. He would keep the fire stoked and put three pieces of spring salmon steak on each stick, cooking them until they were juicy and browned, dripping fat down the sticks. This is still my favourite way to eat salmon. It requires effort and work, but is worth every morsel. I also learned to cook salmon this way.

Fish and Chips

Fish:

    8 pieces sole, individually frozen
    2 C gluten-free corn flakes (honey or plain)
    ¾ C soy, almond, or coconut milk
    olive oil for frying

Chips:

    4 large-sized potatoes
    2 T olive oil
    2 T salt for soaking potatoes
    1 T sea salt, paprika, or MSG-free Hy's Seasoning Salt
    water to cover potatoes

Note: Gluten-free corn flakes can be purchased at Save-On-Foods, Superstores, natural foods stores, and most other grocery stores in the "Gluten-Free" section. I usually grind an entire large bag of corn flakes, then use a bit at a time in a bowl for dredging the fish. For the chips, you can use Idaho, white, or Yukon Gold potatoes. Choose whatever seasoning you prefer.

Preheat oven to 400 to 425 degrees.

Grind the corn flakes in a food processor. Then place 1 cup of ground corn flakes in a flat dish Put the soy, almond, or coconut milk in a bowl. Take one piece of fish and dip in the milk to soak before dredging it in the corn flakes. Then, fry the fish in olive oil for about 30 seconds per side, or until golden brown. You can judge based on what temperature you have set your stove burners.

I usually estimate two pieces of fish per person, but find my family members fighting over this at dinner, as it is so popular—they love this dish!

For the chips, cut the potatoes into slices. Put them in a large bowl of water, add about 2 tablespoons of salt, and soak for about 20 minutes or more. This removes a lot of starch, which allows the chips to bake up crispier and makes them less heavy for those watching their diets. Remove the potato slices from the water, rinse, and pat dry. Coat them with olive oil and seasoning.

Line a large cookie sheet or jelly roll pan with parchment paper. Place the chips in the pan and bake for about 45 minutes. They will be crispy and yummy like the fried version, but healthier and without the calories! Make lots—they will not last!

Preparation time: 20 minutes
Cooking time: 1 minute per piece of sole
Baking time: 45 minutes for the chips
Yield: 4 servings
Serving size: 1 C chips and 2 pieces fish
Calories per serving: 599

Broth

6 to 8 lbs bones, knuckles or joints (3 kg)
4 bay leaves
2 T salt
2 T savoury
1 clove garlic, with outer husk removed
1 large-sized onion, cut into quarters
1 T pepper
fennel (or anise), cut into large pieces
Herbamare
water to cover bones in pot (approximately 32 cups)

Note: I use the bones from any animals we have hunted or from meat obtained from the butcher. In my opinion, bison meat and large marrow bones make the best soup.

Preheat oven to 350 degrees. Take the bones and place them on a pan with the onions and garlic and roast in the oven for about 40 minutes. Take the bones out of the oven. They should be browned and roasted.

Place the roasted bones in a large stockpot with a sieve, and fill the pot with water, covering the bones. Put more onion and garlic, the fennel (or anise), and the remaining herbs and spices in the pot and bring it to a boil.

Once boiling, reduce the heat to a simmer and leave to cook for 24 to 36 hours. This allows all the ingredients to mix together to create an amazing broth. When done, this recipe makes a wonderful broth for soups, gravies, stews, and whatever else you wish to use it for.

I have not bought an over-the-counter broth for over a year now, since I started making my own. I get rave reviews on my homemade soups and stews—especially my bison soup!

Preparation time: 60 minutes
Cooking time: 24 hours
Yield: 32 cups broth
Serving size: 1 cup
Calories per serving: 130

Bison Soup

10 C broth
5 stalks celery, chopped
3 T Herbamare
2 onions, finely chopped
2 C wild rice
1 lb ground bison
1 medium-sized fennel, finely chopped
1 clove garlic, chopped
½ lb organic carrots, chopped
½ lb frozen organic edamame
1/3 C Kloshe Sapolill house blend (optional)
salt to taste
pepper to taste
frozen peas

Note: Add the Kloshe Sapolill is you desire a thicker soup. If you add cooked wild rice, you don't need to do so until later, right near the end, just prior to serving. If you add uncooked wild rice, then do so right at the beginning to allow it to cook all day. As wild rice takes over 45 minutes to an hour to cook on its own, within a soup it will take longer because it is cooking along with the other ingredients.

Place all ingredients in a large pot. Cover with the broth. Or if you use a slow cooker then principal is the same cover with broth. The only change is the slow cooker will take a minimum of 6 hours to cook thoroughly.

Use whatever meat you like. I use either stew meat or ground bison. If I use stew meat, I will fry it in a pan first with olive oil, garlic, and onion until it has browned. Next, I will add about 1/3 cup of Kloshe Sapolill to soak up the fat, and then transfer this mixture to the broth. I always make sure to scrape up the pan afterward.

Once this is done, I will add a well-mixed blend of a cup of Kloshe Sapolill and a cup of broth, stirring this into the pot until everything is thoroughly blended. Then I let the soup cook all day. This allows all the flavours to marinate and mingle.

If you choose to add other items to your soup that require liquid to cook, such as lentils or beans, be sure to use more broth to accommodate these ingredients. Of course, as a highly customizable dish, your soup will be as unique as the ingredients you decide to make it with. Enjoy!

Preparation time: 15 minutes
Cooking time: 1 hour to 6 depending on whether a slow cooker is used.
Yield: 15 cups
Serving size: 1.5 cups
Calories per serving: 210

CHICKEN SOUP

2 lbs chicken (parts or leftover carcass from a roast chicken)
1 to 2 bay leaves
1 clove garlic, halved
1 medium-sized onion, quartered
½ t pepper
½ t poultry seasoning
½ t sage
½ t salt
¼ fresh fennel, quartered
water to cover

Place the roast chicken carcass or chicken parts in a large pot that will hold about 20 cups of water. A Dutch oven works well. Add all ingredients. Cover with water and bring to a boil. Turn the heat down and simmer for 2 hours. Once cooked, pull the bones and parts out to strain the broth. A clearer broth is achieved by skimming the film of fat off the top of the liquid as it is cooking. The broth can be further clarified by straining it through a strainer or cheesecloth. This broth can be stored and frozen either in jars or ziplock bags, or used for soup immediately.

Chicken soup is a simple meal. It is made by bringing to a boil and then simmering chicken parts and/or bones in water, with a variety of flavouring. The flavour of chicken is most potent when it is simmered in water with salt and only a few vegetables, such as onions, carrots, and celery. Variations on the flavour are gained by adding root vegetables such as parsnip, potatoes, sweet potatos, and celery root; herbs such as parsley and dill; and other vegetables such as zucchini, whole garlic cloves, and tomatoes. Saffron or turmeric is sometimes added as a yellow colourant. Seasonings such as black pepper can be added too. The soup should be brought to a boil in a covered pot and cooked on a very low flame for 1 to 3 hours.

You can also use this recipe to make broth for turkey soup after you have cleaned the carcass from a turkey dinner. The nutritional value of chicken soup can be boosted by adding turkey meat to it, as turkey is a richer source of iron. Furthermore, a study has determined that, "Prolonged cooking of bone in a chicken soup increases the calcium content of the soup when cooked at an acidic, and not at a neutral pH." Chicken soup is rich in calcium from the bones—the longer the broth is cooked, the more calcium the bones will release.

This recipe makes a wonderful MSG- and yeast-free broth to use for cooking and making soups, or for cooking wild rice.

Preparation time: 10 minutes
Cooking time: 2 hours
Yield: 15 cups
Serving size: 1.5 cups
Calories per serving: 185

Pizza

3 C Kloshe Sapolill house blend
2 T olive oil
1¼ C buttermilk
1 T baking powder
1 egg white
1 T Coconut Sugar
1 T xanthan gum
¼ t garlic powder
¼ t oregano (or basil or Italian seasoning)
¼ t salt

Note: For buttermilk, I use almond milk left to sour for a few minutes with a teaspoon of lemon juice added. For additional suggestions, please see the section titled "Thickeners, Binders, Substitutions, and Other Additions." Also, egg replacer and egg white are fine to use instead of a real egg. Please keep in mind, though, that egg replacer does contain cornstarch, so use caution if you have issues with corn.

Note: for Yeast risen crust substitute the baking powder with 2 T gluten free yeast and take a quarter cup of almond milk out and warm it before adding the yeast to activate it before adding your liquid to dry ingredients, also adding a pinch of coconut sugar will further activte the yeast as well.

Preheat oven to 400 degrees.

In a large bowl, blend all dry ingredients together. Next, mix all wet ingredients together, then blend wet and dry ingredients until the dough forms into a ball.

Divide the dough ball in half and place both portions onto two pans lined with parchment paper. Place another piece of parchment paper on top, and use a rolling pin to roll the dough out flat. Once this is done, take the top layer of parchment paper off. Put the desired toppings on the pizza dough and place it in the oven to cook for 15 to 20 minutes.

This pizza tastes great with Okanagan's soy cheese, which is a soy cheese that melts very well. It is the best option, in my opinion, for those who can't tolerate dairy. I also use Daiya shredded cheese – which is free of casein and soy. Both of these are excellent choices for those with Lactose intolerances.

Preparation time: 15 minutes
Cooking time: 25 minutes
Yield: 2 large pizza crusts
Serving size: 1/16 as each pizza yields approximately 8 pieces
Calories per serving: crust only is 98

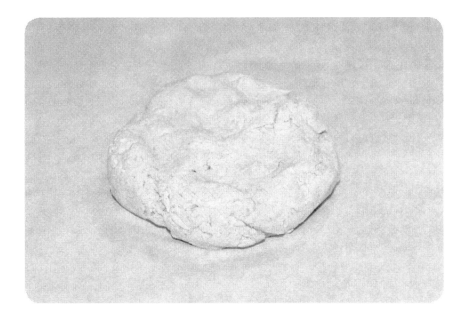

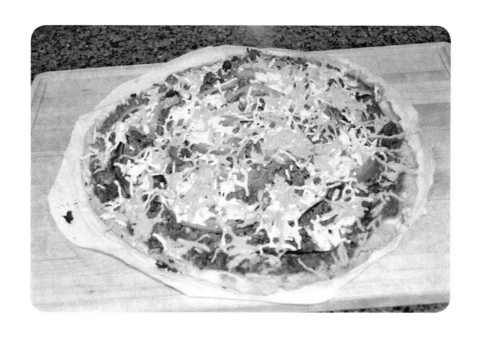

WILD RICE STUFFING

5 to 7 slices any gluten-free bread, chopped into small squares
3 T melted butter
2 C cooked wild rice
1 medium-sized yellow onion, finely chopped
½ t Himalayan sea salt
¼ t pepper
1 clove crushed garlic
poultry seasoning, fresh or dried
water to moisten

Note: In my home, we use Cocolithic bread, a favourite we buy from Just Pies bakery in Penticton, British Columbia. This happens to be the only bread we can use. Also, I like to use poultry seasoning made with about 3 tablespoons of a finely chopped combination of fresh rosemary and thyme.

Preheat oven to 350 degrees. Place the bread, wild rice, garlic and onion in a bowl. Mix the spices and poultry seasoning separately. Add the melted butter to the spice and seasoning mix and blend well. Then add this to the bread, wild rice, and onion combination and mix thoroughly. Moisten this mixture with water.

Take the mixture and stuff it into the bird until the cavity is full. If there is any leftover stuffing once this is done, you can put it into a foil bag and place it in the pan to cook with the bird in the oven. The rule of thumb when cooking a large bird is 13 minutes per pound, so if you have a 15-pound turkey, the total cooking time would be 3 hours and 25 minutes.

You can also choose not to stuff the turkey. In this case, place the stuffing in a pan to cook on its own 35 minutes prior to finishing preparing dinner. It will be ready in time for serving. The method I choose is to soak a turkey in a saltwater brine overnight and then cook the turkey without stuffing it. I cook the stuffing separately, 30 minutes prior to serving dinner.

Preparation time: 20 minutes
Cooking time: varies depending on turkey
Yield: up to 8 servings
Serving size: ¾ cup
Calories per serving: 244

Teaching

I steam my vegetables, which are organic in most cases. Though the cost is slightly higher, going organic is always a choice. My family and I live in the Fraser Valley, where the vegetables are often reasonably priced when in season. Buying from local farmers means that you can purchase vegetables throughout the growing season at a fair price, and then buy organic at your regular grocery store during the off-season. This factors into what cooking and meal planning is all about. I often think about what meals to prepare days in advance. Figuring out what to feed my family is something I think about all the time, as my household is driven by food!

FRIED WILD RICE

10 mini carrots, finely chopped

6 to 7 C water

3 stalks celery, finely chopped

3 C wild rice

2 cloves crushed garlic

2 C cooked quinoa

2 T olive oil

1 large-sized yellow onion, finely chopped

1 t salt

½ C dried cranberries (optional)

½ t Himalayan sea salt

1/3 C chopped walnuts (optional)

¼ C cilantro, finely chopped

¼ of a medium sized fresh fennel, finely chopped

¼ t pepper

Put the wild rice, water, and salt in a large, heavy saucepan and bring it to a boil. Reduce this to a simmer and cook for 45 to 55 minutes, or until the rice seeds open up and the rice looks like it has completely "popped" and the inner whites are visible.

Put all the remaining ingredients in a large, heavy wok and sauté them until they are tender and the flavours mingle. Then add the cooked wild rice and quinoa. Allow everything to mix. Sometimes, I will add a teaspoon of fresh or 1/3 teaspoon of ground turmeric as well, just to give this dish an antifungal boost. I often omit the cranberries due to allergy problems in my home, but they do taste amazing in this recipe. There are many alternatives. This is the favourite with my family.

Preparation time: 15 minutes

Cooking time: 45 minutes for wild rice and 15 minutes additional time for frying

Yield: 15 servings

Serving size: 1.5 C

Calories per serving: 99

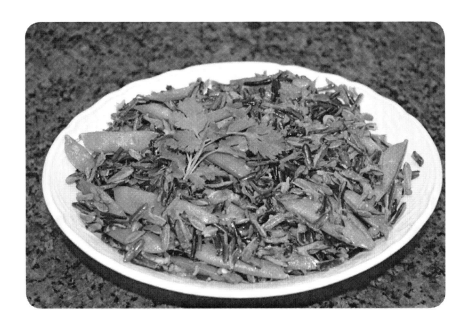

Story Time

When I first met Ken, we used to get together to eat in the lunchroom at work. He would bring his lunch bag . . . and it would have almost the same thing every day. Wild rice, meat, and veggies. There would be a huge amount of each. One day he came in to have lunch and had made this fried wild rice. It was delicious, so we started adding different things to it. Nowadays we add ground meat, diced-up chicken, stew meat, and whatever leftovers we have. It became a staple in our diets and remains so. He cannot eat them, but I like adding dried cranberries to it. So if you can, try this dish with this option—you will love the little bit of sweetness it adds.

MAC 'N' CHEESE

2 C uncooked gluten-free pasta
2 T Kloshe Sapolill house blend (heaping)
2 T margarine
1½ C almond milk (unsweetened)
1½ C shredded Okanagan's soy cheese

Note: A good corn-based pasta is Mrs. Leeper's macaroni, or Presidents Choice which is a housebrand of Superstore and available at all local grocery stores. Also, the total preparation time for this dish can be cut to 20 minutes if the pasta is cooked while you are making the sauce.

Melt the margarine in a medium-sized saucepan on the stove at a temperature of 6 to 7, or medium. Add the Kloshe Sapolill and stir until everything is blended. Use a whisk to ensure this mixture is creamy. Continuously stir it to make sure that there is no clumping. Add the almond milk gradually until it has fully blended. Add the shredded cheese and mix until it has melted and is well blended.

Place a large Dutch oven on the stove filled with about 6 cups of water, and bring it to a full, rolling boil. Add the pasta and reduce the heat to medium. Cook the pasta for about 6 to 8 minutes, until it is al dente. Drain the pasta and rinse it with cool water. Put the pasta back into the Dutch oven and pour the cheese sauce over it.

This gluten-free cheese sauce is lower in calories and milder in taste than the regular version. Though it does taste different, in my household the kids enjoy it, and their friends, from children to teenagers, have all agreed that it is really good. There are never any leftovers! I have used Mrs. Leeper's pasta and wild rice pasta brands. Both are available at Save-On-Foods and

Superstores, as well as at natural foods stores. The prices are not unreasonable. I do find that you need to use Okanagan's soy cheese for the sauce, as it melts well and works best. So do not substitute anything else for this in terms of soy cheese, because the other brands are not reliable for this recipe. Enjoy!

Preparation time: 5 minutes to boil water
Cooking time: 20 minutes for sauce
6 to 8 minutes for pasta
Yield: 4 servings
Serving size: 1½ cups
Calories per serving: 372

Teaching

Living gluten free requires reading everything and understanding what additives are in the foods you eat. It takes hours of research to determine whether there are additives that contain gluten or other items that may cause an allergic reaction. Not all gluten-free products are truly gluten free. The fewer ingredients there are, the more likely it is not to have a reaction. Watch out for "natural flavours"—they tend to be full of chemically altered facsimiles of a flavour, or additives such as organic material and fillers.

BANNOCK

4 C Kloshe Sapolill house blend
4 T baking powder
4 t xanthan gum
1½ C warm water
1 t salt
½ C shortening

Preheat oven to 350 degrees. Line a cookie sheet with parchment paper.

Mix together the flour, baking powder, xanthan gum, and salt until well blended. Cut in the shortening until well blended. I like to use Earth Balance Shortening. It is a vegan product and is essentially a "healthy" fat.

Add warm water until the dough is sticky and forms into a moist ball. Remember that gluten-free dough needs to be moist and sticky to the touch. This is normal.

Take the dough and place on the cookie sheet, flattening it into round bannock "pancakes" about 1 inch thick. Poke fork holes in it a few times.

Place the flattened dough in the oven for about 25 minutes. Remove and cool on the cookie sheet for about 10 minutes prior to transferring it to a wire rack. You can try frying this bread in Coconut oil. With a small amount in pan for frying. The calorie count here is for baking only.

This is a true-blue, gluten-free, and healthy recipe!

Preparation time: 10 minutes
Baking time: 25 minutes

Yield: 12 servings
Serving size: 1 piece 128g
Calories per serving: 342

FLAKY BUTTERMILK BISCUITS

5 T shortening
4 t baking powder
4 T butter, cut into bits
3 C Kloshe Sapolill house blend
1½ C buttermilk
1½ t xanthan gum
1 t salt
1 t coconut sugar

Note: For buttermilk, I use almond milk left to sour for a few minutes with a teaspoon of lemon juice added. For additional suggestions, please see the section titled "Thickeners, Binders, Substitutions, and Other Additions."

Preheat oven to 425 degrees. Grease a baking sheet or line one with parchment paper.

In a medium bowl, combine all dry ingredients and use a whisk to blend thoroughly. Using a pastry blender, cut in the butter and shortening until the mixture is coarse and crumbly. Add the buttermilk and stir just until the dry ingredients are moistened.

Drop ¼-cup mounds of dough about 2 inches apart on the greased or parchment-lined baking sheet. Bake for about 10 to 12 minutes, or until golden brown.

Remove the biscuits from the oven and let them cool slightly. Serve them warm.

These biscuits are like the melt-in-your-mouth regular biscuits, but just a healthier, gluten-free version. They can be served with soy cheese unless you can tolerate regular cheese.

Preparation time: 10 minutes
Baking time: 10 to 12 minutes
Yield: 10 biscuits
Serving size: 135g
Calories per serving: 203

Hamburger and Hotdog Buns

Dry Ingredients:

3 t stevia

2 C + 1 T Kloshe Sapolill house blend

2 t xanthan gum

1 T baking powder

1 t dough improver (optional)

1 t salt

¼ C whey protein

Wet Ingredients:

1¼ C warm water

1 egg white

1 T yeast

¼ C oil (olive, coconut, etcetera)

Note: This recipe contains yeast. For the dough improver recipe, see "Thickeners, Binders, Substitutions, and Other Additions" section.

Preheat oven to 350 degrees.

Mix all dry ingredients in a large bowl. Add the wet ingredients and stir to form a batter.

Line a baking pan with parchment paper. Drop the batter onto the parchment paper, leaving space for it to spread while baking. Once you add the wet ingredients, it is important to get this into the oven immediately. This is in order to benefit from the leavening process, which gives the buns their light and airy feel. Bake for about 20 to 25 minutes.

This versatile recipe is becoming a hamburger and sloppy joe mainstay in my home. It offers a great option for gluten-free eating.

Preparation time: 15 minutes
Baking time: 25 minutes
Yield: 6 buns
Serving size: 115g
Calories per serving: 152

Tortillas

2 C Kloshe Sapolill house blend
2 T shortening
2 t xanthan gum
1½ t salt
1 t baking powder
1 t stevia
1 C warm water

Have a cast-iron flat pan or nonstick cooking pan on hand. A large, flat pan is preferable, as it is similar to a griddle. You can use a tortilla press to make the tortillas a uniform shape and thickness or use a good rolling pin to achieve thickness desired.

Turn on the heat to between 6 and 7, or almost to the maximum temperature, to ensure that the pan gets hot.

In a large bowl, add all dry ingredients and cut in the shortening. Add the warm water slowly until the dough becomes smooth.

Form the dough into balls roughly the size of tennis balls. Place the dough balls on a piece of parchment paper, and then place another piece of parchment on top. Roll the dough out until each ball is flat and circular. Each tortilla's thickness should be about ¼ inch for consistency.

Remove the top piece of parchment paper and turn the tortillas onto the hot pan. Then, remove the other piece of parchment.

Preparation time: 20 minutes
Cooking time: 30 minutes

Yield: 6 servings
Serving size: 125g
Calories per serving: 170

HISTORICAL POINTS OF INTEREST

Regarding the introduction of molasses to the Squamish people, Chief August Jack conveyed this story to Major J. S. Matthews:

"Then Whitemans on schooner give molasses . . . Indian not know what it for, so Indian rub on leg (thighs and calves) for medicine. You know Indian sit on legs for long time in canoe; legs get stiff. Rub molasses on legs make stiffness not so bad. Molasses stick legs bottom of canoe. Molasses not much good for stiff legs, but my ancestors think so. Not their fault, just mistake; they not know molasses good to eat." And then August Khatsahlano laughed heartily.

SWEET

PANCAKES

2 C Kloshe Sapolill house blend
2 egg whites
2 t olive oil
1½ C almond milk
1½ t baking powder
¼ t salt
1 t Cinnamon

Note: If you prefer sugar in your mix, add a tablespoon to it prior to blending.

Blend all ingredients together with a stick blender in a large measuring cup. (I suggest using a 10-cup measuring cup in order to pour your batter onto the griddle as you cook the pancakes.)

Place the griddle on the burners. Use one of those large griddles that covers two burners on the stove. Make sure it is either nonstick or cast iron. Turn the burners on to just around medium to high to bring the temperature up to hot on the griddle. Put some olive oil on the griddle.

Pour the mix so that each pancake is about 3 inches across. This will make approximately four to six pancakes on the griddle per batch.

When the pancakes are bubbling on top, flip them over for about 2 to 3 minutes per side. They will not be really brown because gluten-free pancakes do not brown the same as regular pancakes. They will, however, be fluffy and sugar free.

Variations: Add a mashed banana or ½ C chocolate chips. You can add 1 C Fresh or frozen blueberries as well.

Enjoy! These pancakes are perfect for breakfast or brunch. If any are left over, they are also great for sandwiches later in the day.

Serve these pancakes with my strawberry sauce for a really special treat! If preferred, add maple syrup too.

Preparation time: 10 minutes
Cooking time: 15 minutes
Yield: 12 to 15 medium-sized pancakes
Serving size: 119g
Calories per serving: 123

Story Time

I call these "roadhouse pancakes." Ken was on a road trip with Riel to Manitoba and texted me saying he needed a recipe for pancakes. I had nothing, so I jumped online immediately, piecing together recipes while making them in the kitchen as I texted him the ingredients! We fine-tuned our recipe to come up with these wonderful sugar-free pancakes. In fact, the picture here is one that Ken texted me from his cousin's house in Fisher Branch, Manitoba. This is also where Ken learned that altitude and air pressure made a huge difference in the amount of liquid and cooking temperature affected cooking. There was a need to change the liquid he used in making his pancakes for every province he travelled through. We developed the recipe while he was in Alberta, and he went from there to Saskatchewan and Manitoba. It was a lesson in science and experimentation for both of us.

STRAWBERRY SAUCE

½ bag frozen strawberries (approximately 1 kg)
¼ C stevia
4 t tapioca crystals

Note: Try using whatever fresh fruit is in season and adjust the tapioca crystals to thicken!

Place all ingredients in a large Dutch oven on the stove.

Adjust the temperature to medium heat. Bring the fruit to a boil, and then lower the temperature to a simmer once the fruit heats up. Stir and let the fruit break down. I use a potato masher sometimes to help the fruit reduce completely.

This makes a rich sauce that is very yummy served with my pancakes. If the berries are started just before making the pancakes, everything should be ready at the same time.

Note: we do not use stevia or any other sweetener in the strawberry sauce we make!

Preparation time: 5 minutes
Cooking time: 25 minutes for frozen fruit
15 minutes for fresh fruit
Yield:4 cups
Serving size: ¼ cup per 2 pancakes
Calories per serving: 16.5 and note if you use no
stevia then the calorie count will decrease.

Teaching

Sugar is not required in all foods—we fool ourselves into thinking we need to have sugar in everything we eat because we have grown up with a taste for it. Whipped cream, for example, does not require sugar; we add sugar just to make it sweeter. When we start eating food without sugar, we realize we don't need it. Fresh fruit are a perfect example: their natural sugars are enough. When I cook fruit, their own sugars often provide enough flavour. I will sometimes add small amounts of stevia, a natural plant-based sweetener, to bump it up. But most of the time, this is not necessary. Next time, read the labels on anything in the grocery store. Almost everything has sugar in it and does not need any extra.

Squamish Bars

This recipe is an altered version of Naniamo bars and very delicsious – it is also expensive to make but worth every penny. I found a recipe and altered it to fit for our needs those without gluten intolerances claim it is better!. This is a no bake recipe and uses only the food processor and blender to make this.

Crust:

1.5 C unsweetened coconut
1.5 C Hazelnut or Almond flour*
½ C Coconut Oil melted
¾ C Coconut Sugar (Palm or organic)
¼ C Cocoa or raw cocoa powder
10 dates pitted
2 pinches of sea salt

Filling:

2 C or 2 packages Coconut Cream (*this product comes in a brick form and is just dried coconut meat)
½ C water
½ C maple syrup or coconut nectar
2 tsp Vanilla powder or Vanilla extract **
½ C Melted Coconut Oil
pinch of sea salt

Chocolate topping:

½ C Maple syrup
½ C Coconut oil

½ C Cocoa powder
1 tsp Vanilla Powder or Vanilla Extract

I use whole nuts and grind them into a flour in the food processor – I find this is a less expensive option and you use the nuts you wish to have to flavour the crust for this wonderful recipe

★★ Vanilla powder is in its organic form of ground vanilla bean and has no additives. I do use vanilla extract but only the organic and with no sugar. The only problem with it is it contains alcohol and I prefer the vanilla powder for all recipes.

9 x 9 inch bar pan

In food processor grind the nuts for flour first and add all ingredients for the crust together. Blend in food processor until a paste like consistency about 20 seconds and up to one minute.

scrape the ingredients into the 9 x 9 inch bar pan and place in fridge for about an hour or freezer for about 10 minutes

Place all ingredients for filling in blender and blend at high speed for about 2 minutes or until the entire contents are a creamy consistency. Pour this over the chilled crust and spread until evenly covering the entire pan. Let this cool in fridge for about 1 hour or in freezer for about 10 minutes. The layer should feel firm to touch in middle of pan.

Take all ingredients for Chocolate topping and put in small blender – I like to use my magic bullet or single serving blending cup. Blend ingredients until a smooth chocolate mixture is done this should take about 20 seconds. Pour and scrape the contents on top of the middle custard layer and spread until evenly distributed.

Chill in fridge for about 10-15 minutes or until top layer is firm. Use a bar cutter to make squares in pan into 1.5 inch squares. This makes about 30 squares. They are very rich and feel free to make larger squares. This freezes really well and should be refridgerated as it will melt if left out. This treat is best served chilled.

Preparation time: 45 minutes
Refridgeration time: 2- 3 hours
Yield: 30 squares
Serving size: 1.5 inch squares
Calories per serving:224

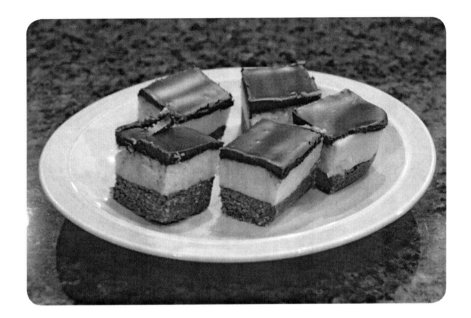

COFFEE CAKE

Cake:

3 C + 1 T Kloshe Sapolill house blend

3 t xanthan gum

2 t baking powder

2 egg whites

2 t organic vanilla extract

1½ C buttermilk

1¼ C softened butter (20 T equivalent)

1 t baking soda

1 t salt

1 C stevia

Topping:

1 T cinnamon

¾ C nuts (your choice; I used walnuts)

½ C stevia (or coconut sugar)

Note: For buttermilk, I use almond milk left to sour for a few minutes with a teaspoon of lemon juice added. For additional suggestions, please see the section titled "Thickeners, Binders, Substitutions, and Other Additions."

Preheat oven to 350 degrees. Line a 13" x 9" x 2" baking pan with parchment paper.

Mix all dry ingredients together in a large bowl. Add softened butter and mix until crumbly. Remove 1 cup of mixture and set aside.

Mix all wet ingredients together. Add wet ingredients to the dry and mix well, until a smooth batter forms. Pour the mixture into the parchment-lined baking dish.

Mix the topping ingredients together in a small bowl and add the reserved 1-cup crumb mixture to this. Sprinkle it on top of the cake evenly and place in the oven to bake for about 50 to 60 minutes, or until toothpick comes out clean.

Preparation time: 20 minutes
Baking time: 50 to 60 minutes
Yield: 12 servings
Serving size: 147g
Calories per serving: 469

Story Time

Ken and Riel are always bugging me for sweets. They wanted coffee cake they could eat, and it was a challenge to come up with the perfect recipe! Do you know just how hard it is to find a coffee cake that is gluten free and almost sugar free? Well, here it is! This coffee cake is pretty good, if I say so myself! Ken and Riel enjoy it made with stevia, but this can be substituted with coconut sugar too. So experiment. I always do!

Cinnamon Buns

Part 1:

3 C Kloshe Sapolill house blend
2 packages quick-rise yeast
¾ C coconut sugar
¾ C softened butter
¼ C xanthan gum

Part 2:

6 eggs (or egg whites)
6 to 10 C flour (depending on need)
water to make 3 cups liquid (lukewarm)

Filling:

3 T cinnamon
2 to 3 C coconut sugar
1¼ C butter

Icing:

4 T cream cheese
3 C icing sugar
2 T butter
1 t organic vanilla extract

Note: This recipe is not sugar free or yeast free.

Preheat oven to 350 degrees. Line two 13" x 9" x 2" pans with parchment paper.

Mix together all ingredients in part one and blend well. Set aside.

Mix together all ingredients in part two. Add this to part one, and then add flour as required until the mixture forms a wet, sticky dough. It should form a dough that is tacky and can be rolled out onto parchment paper to about a ¾-inch thickness. You will need a large surface area for rolling out this dough. I suggest working on a large counter.

Knead the dough and place it in a bowl to rise for about 1 to 1½ hours. It should double in size.

Melt the butter, and add the coconut sugar and cinnamon to it.

Take the dough and place it on a floured surface. Roll it out to about a ¾-inch thickness. You can also use parchment paper to ease the rolling.

Pour the butter, coconut sugar, and cinnamon filling mixture onto the dough surface and spread it around with a spatula until the dough is evenly covered—this is sticky business!

Start carefully rolling the dough at one end until the buns are completely rolled into a large log. Cut into the log to create buns about 1½ inches thick, and then place them in the parchment-lined pans about a ½ inch apart to give them space to expand.

Allow the buns to rise for about 30 minutes. Bake them for about 30 to 45 minutes. This is a good time to combine all ingredients for the icing.

When the buns have doubled in size and browned, they are ready. Remove them from the oven, and allow them to cool for about 10 minutes. Put the icing on top. They can also be enjoyed without it.

Preparation time: 30 minutes
Resting time: 30 minutes for first rising, 30 minutes for second rising
Baking time: 25 minutes
Yield: 18 buns

Serving size: 337g
Calories per serving: 715

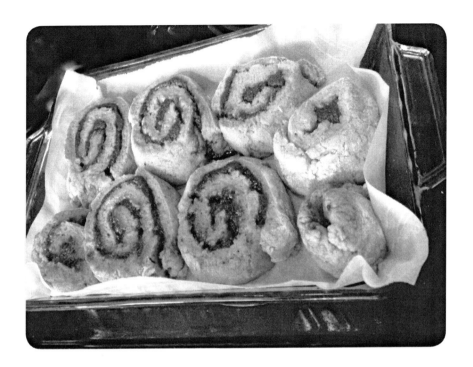

Story Time

These cinnamon buns are a creation I came up with years ago when commercial cinnamon bun shops first arrived on the scene. I craved these ooey, gooey delights, so I fiddled around with a Ukrainian sweet bread recipe until I got the right bun mixture using regular flour. Back then, my original filling mixture contained demerara sugar, butter, good-quality cinnamon, and sometimes raisins. These ingredients made for heavenly cinnamon buns! Today, I have revamped my original recipe to make it gluten free, using coconut sugar instead, and it has turned out really well with my

Kloshe Sapolill house blend flour. Friends and family beg me for this recipe whenever I make a batch of buns, so I am sharing it with the world now!

Banana Bread

4 egg whites
4 C Kloshe Sapolill house blend
3 t xanthan gum
2½ t baking soda
2 t cinnamon
2 t organic vanilla extract
1¾ C mashed bananas (3 to 5 large and overripe)
1 C coconut sugar
1 t salt
¾ C buttermilk
¾ C softened butter

Note: For buttermilk, I use almond milk left to sour for a few minutes with a teaspoon of lemon juice added. For additional suggestions, please see the section titled "Thickeners, Binders, Substitutions, and Other Additions." Fresh or frozen bananas work fine for this recipe. And egg replacer can be used in lieu of real egg whites—just follow the directions on the package. Please keep in mind, though, that egg replacer does contain cornstarch, so use caution if you have issues with corn. Either apple sauce or chia is a suitable swap for egg whites or egg replacer too.

Preheat oven to 350 degrees. Line two loaf pans with parchment paper.

Mix the Kloshe Sapolill, baking soda, salt, and xanthan gum in a bowl and set aside.

Mix the coconut sugar and butter together, and then add the bananas, egg whites, and buttermilk. Let this sit for about 2 minutes, then add in the cinnamon and vanilla extract and blend until creamy.

Add the dry ingredients to the wet and stir until well mixed.

Pour the batter into the loaf pans and bake in the oven until the loaves rise and are brown, about 55 to 60 minutes.

Cool the loaves for about 5 minutes. Pull them out of the pans and cool them fully prior to cutting them into slices.

This recipe originally also had maraschino cherries, chocolate chips, and walnuts. Feel free to add ¾ cup of each of those ingredients if you wish.

Preparation time: 20 minutes
Baking time: 55 to 60 minutes
Yield: 2 loaves, with about 8 pieces each
Serving size: 132g
Calories per serving: 197

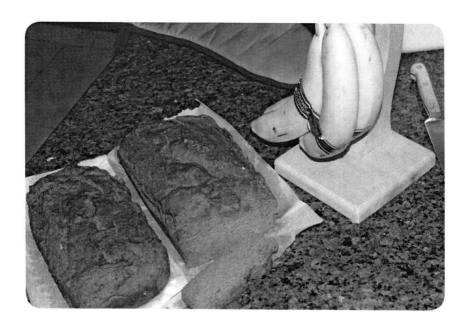

FRESH FRUIT PIE

3 C whole cranberries, fresh or frozen
2 pie crusts (see next recipe)
½ C coconut sugar (or stevia)
¼ C tapioca crystals
pinch of salt

Note: Use whatever fruit you wish. It should be precooked to thicken it prior to filling the pie crust and baking.

Preheat oven to 350 degrees.

Put the fruit in a pot and mix in the tapioca and coconut sugar (or stevia) on low to medium heat. Watch this mixture closely until the fruit breaks down. As the fruit cooks it will thicken, so the temperature should be reduced to a low simmer and then shut off completely. This process takes about 30 minutes.

Roll out one of the pie crust pastries and place it in a pie plate. Take a ladle or large spoon and pour the fruit mixture into the pie crust, but do not overfill it.

Gently apply the second pie crust over the fruit filling. Use a fork to press down the edges of the top crust so that it seals together with the bottom crust. With a knife, pierce the top pie crust.

You can glaze the top crust with a beaten egg and sprinkle it with sugar if desired.

Place the pie in the oven and bake it for about 25 to 30 minutes, until the crust turns golden brown.

Preparation time: 20 minutes
Baking time: 30 minutes
Yield: 1 pie, with about 8 servings
Serving size: 55g
Calories per serving: 142

PIE CRUST

2¼ C + 1 T Kloshe Sapolill house blend
2 T lemon juice
2 T water
1 t baking powder
1½ t xanthan gum
1 egg white
1 t salt
1 T stevia
¾ C vegan lard or shortening

Note: I have used many different types of lards and fats, and I have found through trial and error that the best type is Earth Balance Shortening or the same brand's "butter stick." I use only these because of the allergy issues in my home; they cause the least reactions. You are welcome to use conventional lard as well. Feel free to experiment with different lards or shortenings according to your preferences.

Combine all dry ingredients. Add the lard or shortening and mix until well blended. The consistency should be as pea-like as possible.

Mix all wet ingredients. Add them to the dry ingredients and form a ball of dough.

I use parchment paper to roll out my pastry dough. I place the dough on the paper and put another piece of parchment paper on top of the dough. Then I roll out the dough to the appropriate size and thickness before placing it in the pie plate. This pastry dough is a little more fragile than the regular kind, but it is still very flaky and delicious once baked.

Preparation time: 20 minutes
Yield: Four 9-inch crusts; 2 top, 2 bottom
Serving size: 55g
Calories per serving: 142

REGULAR HOMEMADE PIE CRUST

5 to 6 C flour (gluten free optional)
1 egg
1 lb lard (not shortening)
1 t salt
1 t vinegar
water

Crack the egg into a cup, add the vinegar, and then add enough water to make 1 cup. Mix with a fork vigorously. Set aside.

Pour the flour into a large bowl and add the salt. Cut in the lard. Mix in the lard until the flour feels clumpy. Once the lard is thoroughly blended with the flour, the mixture will have a crumbly, pea-like consistency. Add the egg, vinegar, and water mix. Blend this in with a spoon and then with your hands until a dough is formed. If needed, add more flour until the dough can be formed into a large ball. Knead the dough to make it elastic and even. You do not want it to be sticky, so use flour to make sure it is smooth and pliable.

Cut the dough into 4 smaller balls. Take a ball of dough and split it in half. Roll out one of the halves onto a flour-dusted surface until it is about 1/8 inch thick. Place the rolled-out dough in a 9- or 10-inch pie plate. Place the desired filling in the dough. Cut the excess dough from the edge of the pie plate with a knife. Then take the remaining half of the dough ball and roll it out to make the top crust.

Fold the top dough in half. Use a knife to cut steam holes and place the folded dough on top of your pie filling. Use your finger and thumb to pinch the shell together along the edge of the pie plate (or use a fork to do the same thing). You can use an egg wash on the top pie crust and sprinkle sugar on it before putting it into the oven. This will give the crust a lovely brown finish once it is done baking. This recipe will make enough dough for about four to five large pies.

Preparation time: 20 minutes
Yield: Ten 9-inch crusts; 5 top, 5 bottom
Serving size: 184g
Calories per serving: 290

Story Time

This is the only non-gluten-free recipe in my book, but I included it because it has been the cornerstone of my life for as long as I can remember. It has also been the one thing my entire family still relies on me to bake for them. My granny, Eva, used to make pies and take them to sell at the Mosquito Creek Marina in North Vancouver every week. The money she raised helped feed her family. I asked my mom how to make pies when I was about five years old. She laughed but described the ingredients and the process. I came back from the kitchen a couple of hours later and showed her what I had made. Mom was so impressed she was speechless! So this is a beloved family tradition passed down from dear Granny Eva.

Almond Coconut Tart

Pastry:

Use Pie Crust recipe

Filling:

3 egg whites
2 C unsweetened desiccated coconut
1½ C honey
1 C ground almonds
½ C Kloshe Sapolill house blend
¼ C coconut oil
¼ t salt

Preheat oven to 350 degrees. Roll out the pie crust onto the bottom of a 13" x 9" x 2" pan.

Mix the filling and pour half of it into the pie crust. Put 2/3 of the crumble topping on the syrup.

Place the tart into the oven for 25 minutes, or until it is golden brown.

Take any remaining pie crust and divide it into balls. Wrap them in parchment paper and freeze them until a later time. Take any of the remaining crumble topping and freeze it as well.

This recipe is similar to that of a butter tart. In fact, it is a revised butter tart recipe I have had for over twenty-five years.

Preparation time: 30 minutes
Baking time: 25 minutes
Yield: 15 bars
Serving size: 150g
Calories per serving: 549

Teaching

Cooking and baking are similar to science—experimentation is necessary in order to find what works. The majority of my recipes are old recipes collected over the course of thirty-five years. It is necessary to make adjustments to get the right texture, get the desired taste, and meet the appropriate needs when entering the world of gluten free. We all commonly adjust spices to taste, so recipes with flours are no different. They too require trial and error to achieve success.

CARROT CAKE WITH CREAM CHEESE ICING

Cake:

3 egg whites
2 t baking powder
2 t cinnamon
2 C grated carrots
2 C Kloshe Sapolill house blend
2 t xanthan gum
1½ C stevia
1 t baking soda
1 C drained crushed pineapple
1 t organic vanilla extract
¾ C olive oil
¾ t salt
½ C chopped nuts
½ t nutmeg
Icing:
8 oz cream cheese
3 C icing sugar
1 t organic vanilla extract

Note: You can use whatever oil and nuts you prefer. I use olive oil and walnuts.

Preheat oven to 350 degrees. Grease and flour a 13" x 9" x 2" pan or line it with parchment paper.

In a large bowl, mix together all dry ingredients. In a separate large measuring cup, mix together all wet ingredients. Stir the wet ingredients into the dry ingredients and blend well.

Spread this mixture evenly into your greased or parchment-lined pan. Place it into the oven for about 40 minutes, until the center of the cake is evenly brown or a toothpick comes out clean. Let the cake cool in the pan on a rack before cutting it into squares.

If you would like to serve this cake with cream cheese icing, simply blend the icing ingredients until creamy and spread on top of the cake once it is cool. In my home, we find that this cake is moist enough to eat without icing.

Preparation time: 20 minutes
Baking time: 40 minutes
Yield: 12 servings
Serving size: 181g
Calories per serving: 435

ALL-OCCASION CAKE

3 egg whites
1.5 C Almond or coconut Milk
1t Lemon Juice
1.5 t baking powder
1.5 t Baking Soda
2.75 C Kloshe Sapolill house blend
1 t xanthan gum
1 T organic vanilla extract or vanilla powder
.75 C softened butter
1¼ C Coconut sugar
pinch of salt
.75 C Shortening
Coconut sugar icing
2 C Powdered Coconut Sugar (take regular coconut sugar and
powder it in a food processor for 3 minutes)
1é3 C Butter
1 t vanilla powder
2 – 3 T Coconut milk

Preheat oven to 350 degrees. Line bottom of a spring form pan with parchment paper, snap the base back in place with parchment paper sticking out of bottom of pan.

In a large mixing bowl, mix together all wet ingredients and the coconut sugar. In a separate measuring cup, mix together all dry ingredients.

Blend the dry ingredients in with the wet and mix with an electric mixer for 2 minutes, scraping the sides of the bowl to ensure proper blending.

Scrape the batter into the parchment-lined pan and spread it evenly. Place the pan in the oven and bake for 20 to 25 minutes. The cake will turn slightly brown. Remember that gluten-free baked items do not always turn completely brown when ready. So it is important to watch the cake closely. It will be done when it bounces to the touch and a toothpick inserted comes out clean.

Remove the cake from the oven. Allow it to cool in the pan on a rack for 10 minutes before turning it out onto the rack to cool completely and removing the parchment paper.

Decorate the cake with Coconut sugar icing when cake is completely cool..

Preparation time: 20 minutes
Baking time: 25 minutes
Decorating time: 20 minutes
Yield: 10 servings
Serving size: 175g
Calories per serving: 300

Story Time

This recipe has been adjusted from one that used white chocolate and whipped creamfrom a red velvet cake. It was well received at my mother's seventieth birthday, and even she had to admit that it was pretty fabulous! As a diabetic, my mom struggles with eating right, so I used fresh berries on top of the cake and did not add sugar to the whipped cream.

Chocolate cake add 1 third of a cup of cocoa

For Red Velvet cake: 1 third cup cocoa and 3 T Red food colour.

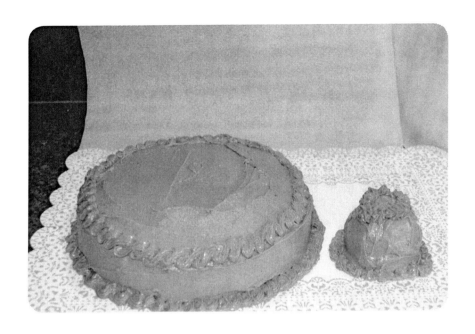

Coconut Power Bars

2 C coconut chips (150 g)
2 C unsweetened desiccated coconut (150 g)
2 egg whites
1 to 1½ C pumpkin seeds
1 C chopped almonds
¾ C coconut oil
¾ C honey (coconut sugar or maple syrup)
¾ C Kloshe Sapolill house blend

Note: If you are not allergic to dried fruit, you can add 1 cup of raisins, dried cranberries, dried blueberries, etcetera to your liking to change up this recipe.

Preheat oven to 350 degrees. Put the coconut oil and sugar or honey or maple syrup in a saucepan and heat until the butter is melted. Take off the heat and leave to cook slightly.

Sift the Kloshe Sapolill into a mixing bowl and add all the remaining ingredients. Stir with a wooden spoon until everything is well blended. Tip the mixture into a prepared tin or pan and press down using the back of a spoon.

Bake in the oven for 20 to 25 minutes, until the top is golden brown and the mixture feels firm to the touch.

Let the mixture cool completely in the tin or pan. Then transfer it onto a chopping board and cut it into bars. These bars keep for up to five days if stored in an airtight container.

Preparation time: 10 minutes
Baking time: 25 minutes
Yield: about 12 bars
Serving size:132g
Calories per serving: 466

HEALING

HERBAL TEAS

Now, this is an area that I normally leave to my baby sister, Cease Wyss—it is her bailiwick, so to speak! She is an authority on tea. I always defer to her knowledge of it as well as her expertise on Native local medicines acquired through more than twenty-five years of vast travel and research. So I apologize for the modest information presented here, but please be on the lookout for our future collaborations on cookbooks as well as on food, beverage, and medicinal guides.

Brew your own soothing infusion with the help of this guide to herbal teas. These concoctions offer pleasant alternatives for tea drinkers who want to avoid caffeine. They also help relieve common health discomforts.

CHAMOMILE

A mild sedative, chamomile tea is said to aid digestion and relieve menstrual cramps. Trace amounts of pollen residue in chamomile tea may cause dermatitis or other allergic symptoms in people sensitive to ragweed, chrysanthemums, and members of the daisy family.

DANDELION

Tea made from this common weed is mildly diuretic. Some women use it to reduce premenstrual bloating.

ELDERFLOWER

Extracts of elder are sometimes used in over-the-counter cold remedies, and elderflower tea may alleviate cold and flu symptoms. Elderflowers and ripe elderberries are safe, but avoid the roots, stems, and leaves. The tea is also a mild stimulant.

FENNEL

With a flavour similar to licorice, fennel tea is used to soothe an upset stomach. Traditional herbalists often recommend it as an appetite suppressant and slimming aid.

LABRADOR

Still found in bogs, the Labrador plant's aromatic young twigs, leaves, and flowers have long been used both fresh and dried for tea. It is a good medicine for colds and sore, irritated throats. The tea should be weak; a small handful of leaves steeped in boiling water for five minutes yields a pleasant beverage.

LAVENDER FLOWER

Tea brewed from dried lavender flowers is said to be a mild sedative.

LEMON BALM

This minty tea may help soothe jittery nerves.

NETTLE

Made from the same plant that causes stinging skin irritation, nettle tea is rich in vitamin C and several minerals. Herbalists recommend it to treat arthritis and gout, and to increase milk production in nursing mothers.

Peppermint

Tea from this mint plant is refreshing and may stimulate digestion. It should, however, be avoided by anyone with a hiatal hernia, because peppermint promotes reflux of the stomach contents into the esophagus.

Raspberry Leaf

Herbalists recommend raspberry leaf tea to ease menstrual cramps.

Rose Hip

Rich in vitamin C, rose hip tea can substitute as an alternative to orange juice.

Rosemary

Tea from this popular garden herb is said to relieve gas and colic, but drinking more than two or three cups a day may irritate the stomach.

Thyme

Herbalists recommend thyme tea for gastrointestinal complaints and to alleviate lung congestion.

Squamish elders didn't brew tea and throw away the cooked berries. These were used in soups and stews. The "leftovers," cooked in a largish batch of rose hip tea, are a good dinner vegetable with butter and salt (the berries expand a lot). There is still a lot of remaining food value in the cooked berries.

Story Time

My family and I like to go to North Vancouver to the Harmony Garden, a community garden built in the heart of the Capilano Reserve on Squamish Nation land. It is the brainchild of my sister and mother. They approached the band and asked for permission to use a deserted piece of land that people were utilizing as a garbage dump. Soon this area was transformed into a thriving community garden to support the community kitchen my mother and sister created at St. Paul's Church in North Vancouver to feed people with little or no access to good, nutritional food. This kitchen has been in operation for over ten years now, and the community garden is in its fifth year. Harmony Garden provides many of the fresh vegetables and herbs used by the community kitchen, as well as indigenous medicines and berries. During my family's past few visits, my children have worked in the garden in the summertime, earning a little cash and a lot of experience. They have also partaken in beekeeping the last two years. We are always guaranteed a pot of tea made with fresh picks from the garden my sister has put together, including berries, herbs, and natural medicines. These experiences are always a wonderful treat.

Bibliography

Davis, William. *Wheat Belly: Lose the Wheat, Lose the Weight, and Find Your Path Back to Health.* Emmaus, Pennsylvania: Rodale Press, 2011.

Junger, Alejandro. Clean Gut: The Breakthrough Plan for Eliminating the Root Cause of Disease and Revolutionizing Your Health. San Francisco: HarperOne, 2013.

Matthews, James Skitt. *Early Vancouver* (vols. 1, 2). Vancouver: City of Vancouver, 2011.

Nahanee, Teressa Ann and Wyss, Barbara. *Inter-Tribal Cookbook: Recipes of North American Indians; Traditional and Modern.* Lone Butte, British Columbia: BRT Publishers, 1982.

Ustlahn Social Society. Berry Cakes: Past and Present Diet of the Squamish People; A Story of Food and Cultural Change over 200 Years. North Vancouver: Ustlahn Social Society, 2010.

http://www.doctoroz.com/videos/surprising-health-benefits-coconut-oil

Used for research on oils and fats.

http://nutritiondata.self.com
Used for research on nutritional data for recipes.

http://www.sparkpeople.com
Used for research on nutritional data for recipes.

http://en.wikipedia.org/wiki/main_page
Used for research on flours, sugars, and gums.

http://www.wisegeek.com
Used for research on flours and grains.

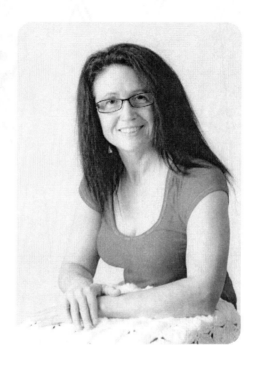

I am Yvonne Bonnie Wyss. Born in Vancouver and grew up in the Province of British Columbia Canada. I am a "West Coast" Girl as my partner likes to refer to me - as he is from the Prairies and among first nations people we identify ourselves by regions and nations often. I grew up mainly in the Lower mainland near Vancouver British Columbia. My background and education is in Administration and nursing.

My four children and I live with my Partner and his son who provided me with the inspiration to create this book. because of his allergies and perspectives on food, I also had many health issues over the years. We discovered that other people where interested in how we have chosen to live a Gluten free lifestyle.

I am a cultural person who has strong cultural and spiritual ties to my own Longhouse people whom I descend from as well as the The prairie cultural and spiritual path I follow in my own life.

I personally believe in what I do with passion and my book is shared from the heart to offer my own personal journey. I lost nearly 60lbs by changing my life for this.

byvonne@shaw.ca

www.YBGlutenFree.ca

CPSIA information can be obtained at www.ICGtesting.com
Printed in the USA
LVOW11s0048090714

393434LV00004B/11/P

9 781460 239766